# How to conduct your own therapy

## Unlock the Power of Self-Healing for a Happier and Healthier You

By

Dr. Raul P. Wheeler

# Table of contents


Copyright

Description

Introduction

Chapter 1

Understanding yourself

Establish a self-care routine

Develop self- awareness

Identify Your Triggers and Cope with Stressors

Chapter 2

Establishing a Safe and Supportive Environment

Identify What You Want to Achieve

Learn Self-Awareness and Self-Regulation

Employ Effective Self-Care Practices

Develop a Support System

Chapter 3

practicing mindfulness

Identify Your Stressors

Observe Your Feelings and Thoughts

Develop Self-Compassion

Establish Self-Care Practices

Chapter 4

Steps to Self-Therapy

Assessing Your Mental Health

Understanding Your Feelings and Thoughts

Developing Coping Mechanisms

Creating a Self-Care Plan

Chapter 5

Ways of Maintaining Self-Therapy

Journaling

Seeking Professional Guidance

Connecting with Others

Conclusion

# Copyright

# Description

Are you tired of feeling stuck and struggling to make progress in life?  Are you feeling overwhelmed and exhausted by the ever-changing circumstances in life? It's time to take control of your life and become your own therapist with the book How to Be Your Own Therapy. This groundbreaking book helps you learn how to be your own therapist and become your own source of support and guidance. With powerful strategies and techniques, this book will enable you to take charge of your mental health and well-being.

You will learn how to build a strong foundation for self-care and create a personalized plan for managing stress, depression, and anxiety. You will gain insight into the power of mindfulness, reframing thoughts, and cognitive-behavioral techniques to help you manage difficult emotions and create lasting change.

You will also learn how to create an action plan, develop healthy habits, and build healthy relationships. This book is packed with practical guidance and techniques to help you take charge of your mental health.

It's time to take control of your life and become your own therapist. Get the book How to Be Your Own Therapy and start your journey to a healthier, happier, and more fulfilling life.

Take the first step towards a healthier and happier life today. Get your copy of How to Be Your Own Therapy and start your journey to mental health and well-being. Order your copy today and start taking control of your life and becoming your own therapist.

# Introduction

Welcome to the world of self-therapy! For many of us, self-therapy is a challenging but rewarding endeavor. It can help us to better understand ourselves, our relationships, and our motivations, and can provide a safe space to explore and grow our emotional, mental, and spiritual health. How to Conduct Your Own Therapy is a comprehensive guide to self-therapy. This book offers a step-by-step approach to help you better understand yourself and develop your inner strength and resilience. It provides an overview of the different types of self-therapy, including meditation, mindfulness, journaling, and self-reflection. It also covers specific techniques to help you access your innermost thoughts and feelings, including guided imagery, visualization, and affirmations.

Whether you are just starting out on your self-therapy journey or have been on it for years, this book provides a valuable resource to help you better understand yourself and your relationships. It offers practical advice on how to make the most of your self-therapy sessions, as well as tips on how to stay motivated and consistent.

Take the first step to understand yourself and your relationships better. This book provides the tools and guidance you need to make self-therapy an effective and rewarding part of your life.

# Chapter 1

## Understanding yourself

Understanding yourself is a key step in becoming your own therapist. It involves taking a deep look at yourself and understanding your unique strengths, weaknesses, and life experiences. It requires you to take the time to reflect on your beliefs and values and to explore how these have shaped your life.

One of the most important aspects of understanding yourself is being aware of your emotions, thoughts, and feelings. It is essential to be able to identify and distinguish between emotions and to be able to manage them effectively. It is also important to be aware of how your emotions and thoughts affect your behavior.

Also, it involves developing a better understanding of your needs and wants. This involves recognizing the needs that are important to you and understanding how these needs can be met healthily and positively. It also involves recognizing and understanding what drives your behavior and the impact that it has on your life.

In addition to being aware of your emotions, thoughts, and feelings, it is also important to understand the impact of your life experiences. This includes understanding how past experiences have shaped your beliefs, values, and behavior. It is also important to understand how certain life experiences can trigger certain emotions, thoughts, and behaviors.

Finally, understanding yourself involves being aware of your unique strengths and weaknesses. This includes recognizing the areas in which you excel and the areas in which you could use improvement. It also involves understanding the areas in which you are most vulnerable and how to best protect yourself.

Understanding yourself is a crucial step in becoming your own therapist. It involves taking the time to understand and reflect on the unique aspects of yourself and how they have shaped your life. This can help you to better understand yourself, your needs, and how to best manage your emotions, thoughts, and behavior.

# Establish a self-care routine

Establishing a self-care routine is one of the best ways to be your own therapist. Self-care is an important part of managing stress and maintaining a healthy mental and physical balance. It can also help to foster feelings of self-compassion, self-love, and connectedness.

A good self-care routine should be tailored to your individual needs. Start by identifying any areas of your life where you may be feeling overwhelmed or lacking in motivation. It could be anything from improving your diet to getting more exercise, to taking some time each day to practice relaxation or mindfulness.

Creating a list of activities that you enjoy will help you to make self-care a part of your daily routine. Consider activities such as reading, listening to music, writing, cooking, or taking a walk. Make sure to also include activities that are specifically designed to reduce stress, such as yoga, meditation, and journaling.

It is also important to make sure that your self-care routine is realistic and achievable. Make sure to set yourself achievable goals and reward yourself for meeting them.

Self-care isn't just about taking care of yourself physically, it's also about taking care of your mental health. Spend time each day reflecting on positive affirmations, and regularly engage in activities that make you feel good.

By creating a self-care routine, you can become your own therapist and learn how to manage stress, reduce anxiety, and cultivate a sense of well-being.

# Develop self- awareness

Self-awareness is an important tool on the path to becoming your own therapist. It involves understanding your thoughts, feelings, and behaviors, and being able to recognize how they interact and influence each other. Self-awareness helps you identify your strengths, weaknesses, and triggers and allows you to understand yourself better so you can make more informed decisions.

One way to develop self-awareness is to practice mindfulness. This involves paying attention to the present moment without judgment and acknowledging your thoughts and feelings without reacting to them. It allows you to observe your thoughts and feelings without getting caught up in them.

Keeping a journal is another method for increasing self-awareness. Writing down your thoughts and feelings can help you identify patterns in your behavior and reactions. It can also help you to recognize your triggers and become more mindful of them.

 It's important to practice self-compassion. This means being kind to yourself and recognizing that your thoughts, feelings, and behaviors are valid, even if they're not ideal. It's critical to keep in mind that you are not flawless and that making mistakes is ok. Developing self-awareness is an important step in becoming your own therapist. By understanding your thoughts, feelings, and behaviors, you can gain insight into what triggers you and how to better manage those triggers. It can help you to make more informed decisions and develop healthier coping mechanisms.

# Identify Your Triggers and Cope with Stressors



Being your own therapist is all about learning to recognize and manage stressors, as well as identify and cope with triggers. Stressors are the external factors in your life that can cause stress, such as work deadlines, financial obligations, and family issues. Triggers are the internal mental, emotional, or physical responses to these stressors. By being aware of your triggers and understanding how to cope with them, you can take control of your mental health.

One way to identify your triggers is to keep a journal and note your thoughts, feelings, and behaviors in response to stress. This will help you become aware of how certain situations or experiences can trigger certain emotional responses. Once you've identified some of your triggers, the next step is to develop effective coping strategies.

Cognitive-behavioral therapy (CBT) is a great way to learn how to cope with stressors and triggers. CBT teaches you to challenge negative thoughts and behaviors and focus on more productive ways of thinking and responding. It also helps you to recognize and understand your own triggers and develop strategies to manage them.

Another way to cope with stressors and triggers is to practice mindfulness. Mindfulness involves being aware of your thoughts and feelings without judgment or criticism. It can help you to recognize your triggers and focus on the present moment, rather than getting caught up in past experiences or worrying about the future.

It's important to take care of yourself and find healthy ways to manage stress. Regular exercise, eating a balanced diet, getting enough sleep, and engaging in activities that bring joy are all great ways to reduce stress and improve your overall well-being.

By taking the time to identify your triggers and learn effective coping strategies, you can become your own therapist and take control of your mental health.

# Chapter 2

## Establishing a Safe and Supportive Environment

Creating a safe and supportive environment for yourself is an important part of being your own therapist. It's important to create a space that allows you to feel comfortable exploring your thoughts and feelings. This could include setting up a designated space in your home or office, like a desk or corner in your bedroom, where you can focus on yourself. You may find it helpful to dedicate a few minutes each day to reflecting on your feelings or writing in a journal.

Creating a supportive environment also means establishing boundaries with yourself. This means setting limits on how much time you spend on self-care activities, as well as what types of activities you engage in. For example, you may want to limit the amount of time you spend on social media or watching television to dedicate more time to self-care. Additionally, it's important to establish a sense of self-compassion and understanding. This means being gentle with yourself and recognizing that it's okay to make mistakes or have difficult days.

It's critical to have a support system in place. This could include family, friends, and mental health professionals who can provide you with guidance and understanding. Additionally, engaging in activities that bring joy and peace can also be a great way to create a supportive environment. This could include activities like yoga, meditation, or simply taking a walk outside in nature.

Creating a safe and supportive environment for yourself is essential when it comes to being your own therapist. Establishing boundaries and self-compassion, as well as having a strong support system, can help you to feel more secure in exploring your thoughts and feelings. Additionally, engaging in activities that bring you joy and peace can help to create a more positive environment.

# Identify What You Want to Achieve

Therapy can be an incredibly helpful tool for managing mental health issues and improving overall well-being. However, it can also be expensive and time-consuming, making it difficult to access for many. Fortunately, there are many ways that one can be their own therapist. Identifying what you want to achieve and taking the initiative to work towards it is the first step.

The most important part of being your own therapist is to identify what you want to achieve. This could include improving your overall mental health, managing a specific mental health issue, or simply feeling better about yourself. Once you have identified what you want to achieve, you can create a plan for yourself to work towards it. This plan should include both short- and long-term goals and should be realistic and achievable.

The next step is to create a self-care routine. Self-care is an important part of being your own therapist and should include activities that both help manage symptoms and cultivate positive feelings. This could include mindful activities such as yoga and meditation, or more creative activities like drawing, writing, and listening to music.

It is important to create an accountability system. This could be a friend or family member that you check in with regularly, or even a therapist if you feel comfortable doing so. Having someone to talk to and discuss your progress with can be incredibly helpful in staying on track and achieving your goals.

Being your own therapist is an empowering experience, and can help you take control of your mental health. Identifying what you want to achieve and creating a plan to work towards it is the first step, and can be done with enough dedication and self-care.

# Learn Self-Awareness and Self-Regulation

Self-awareness and self-regulation are two powerful tools that can help you be your own therapist. Knowing yourself, understanding yourself, and managing your emotions and behavior can lead to a better sense of well-being, improved relationships, and greater success in life. Self-awareness involves having a clear picture of yourself and your goals. It also involves understanding your strengths and weaknesses, motivations, and values. Through self-awareness, you can learn to recognize your needs and feelings and become better at managing your emotions. Self-regulation involves taking the time to practice self-care and build emotional resilience. This includes learning to recognize and manage stress, developing better problem-solving skills, and learning how to set boundaries. Practicing mindfulness and meditation can also help to increase self-regulation.

Being your own therapist requires a commitment to self-reflection and personal growth. It involves learning to recognize and accept areas of weakness, but also to celebrate and cultivate areas of strength. It also involves taking responsibility for your choices, actions, and mistakes.

Being your own therapist requires learning how to regulate emotions and behaviors. This involves understanding when and how to take a break, how to manage stress, and how to practice self-compassion. It also involves learning how to set healthy boundaries and manage relationships.

By learning self-awareness and self-regulation, you can become your own therapist and take charge of your life. With practice, you can become more aware of your needs and feelings, and better able to manage them in healthy, constructive ways.

# Employ Effective Self-Care Practices



Self-care is crucial for general health and happiness. It helps us maintain our physical and mental health, and can even help us cope with difficult situations. Effective self-care involves taking the time to nurture and care for yourself and doing things that make you feel relaxed and balanced.

A key element of effective self-care is understanding your needs and finding ways to meet them. This could include activities such as getting enough rest, eating nutritious meals, exercising regularly, and taking time to relax. It's also important to build healthy relationships with others, as having supportive relationships can help to reduce stress.

Another aspect of self-care is learning to be your own therapist. This involves identifying and addressing your own needs, as well as recognizing the signs of stress and taking steps to manage it. It's important to take time to reflect on your thoughts and feelings and to practice self-compassion and acceptance.

Developing healthy coping skills is also important for self-care. This includes identifying and managing triggers, learning to manage difficult emotions, and using distraction techniques to break negative thought patterns. It's also important to set realistic goals and to recognize and celebrate your successes. Overall, effective self-care helps us to look after our physical and mental health, and to cope with challenging situations. Taking the time to nurture ourselves, understanding our needs, and learning to be our own therapists are all important aspects of effective self-care.

# Develop a Support System

Developing a support system is essential for those who want to be their own therapist. A support system is a collection of people, resources, and activities that provide emotional and practical assistance to someone in need. It is important to have a diverse group of individuals in your support system who can provide you with different perspectives and experiences. Having a support system in place can help you cope with difficult situations and challenges in your everyday life. Friends and family can provide comfort and understanding and can offer emotional support when you're feeling overwhelmed or down. Building strong relationships with people you trust can provide a sense of security and validation. It's also important to have people in your life who are willing to listen, offer advice, and support you in whatever way they can.

It also helps to have access to professional help. A therapist or counselor can provide guidance and support when you're facing difficult issues and can help you process your feelings and move toward positive change. They can also provide referrals to other professionals or resources, such as psychiatric care or support groups.

In addition, seeking out activities and hobbies that you enjoy can help you manage stress and improve your mental health. Exercise, meditation, and creative pursuits such as art, music, or writing can be very therapeutic and can provide a sense of purpose and fulfillment.

Finally, don't forget to take care of yourself. Eating healthy, getting enough sleep, and taking time for yourself are all important for maintaining your mental health. Keep in mind that you are not alone and that asking for assistance when you require it is acceptable. Developing a support system can help you be your own therapist and navigate life's challenges.

# Chapter 3

## practicing mindfulness

Mindfulness is a powerful tool that can help us become our own therapists. It is a practice that helps us to become aware of our thoughts, feelings, and physical sensations in the present moment. Through mindfulness, we can learn to recognize our triggers, observe our reactions without judgment, and find ways to respond in healthier and more compassionate ways.

The first step in becoming your own therapist is to practice mindfulness. This can be done through activities such as mindful meditation, mindful walking, and mindful eating. Mindful meditation involves paying attention to your breath as it moves in and out of your body. Mindful walking involves focusing on your physical sensations and the environment around you. Mindful eating involves paying attention to the taste, texture, and smell of your food.

When practicing mindfulness, it is important to observe your thoughts and feelings without judgment. This means allowing yourself to experience whatever comes up without labeling it as "good" or "bad". This can help you gain insight and understanding into your thoughts and feelings, allowing you to respond to them in healthier ways.

Another important aspect of becoming your own therapist is to practice self-compassion. This means being kind and understanding with yourself when things don't go as planned or when you don't reach your goals. Self-compassion can help you to accept yourself as you are and make healthier choices.

Finally, it is important to remember to be patient with yourself. Becoming your own therapist takes time and patience, and it is important to be gentle with yourself as you go through this process.

Overall, practicing mindfulness can be an effective way to become your own therapist. It can help you to gain insight into your thoughts and feelings and respond to them in healthier ways. It can also help you to practice self-compassion and be patient with yourself. By committing to mindfulness, you can learn to be your own therapist and make healthier choices.

# Identify Your Stressors

Identifying your stressors is an important part of being your own therapist. Stressors are any external factor that can cause distress and can include environmental, physical, and psychological triggers. To successfully identify and manage your stressors, you must first understand what they are and how they impact your life. Environmental stressors can be anything from loud noises to strong odors, and can even include other people. Identifying environmental stressors means paying attention to when and where you feel the most stressed. When you recognize a pattern, try to find ways to reduce or eliminate the stress trigger. This can include wearing earplugs in noisy areas, avoiding heavily-scented places, or limiting your time with certain people. Physical stressors are often related to your body's response to certain stimuli. These can include hunger, fatigue, pain, or even certain medications. To cope with these physical stressors, it's important to maintain a healthy diet and lifestyle and to get enough rest. Additionally, if you are taking any medications, check with your doctor to make sure they are not contributing to your stress.

Finally, psychological stressors are any emotional or mental triggers that can cause distress. These can include worry, fear, or even regret. To identify and manage these stressors, it's important to take time to recognize and process your emotions. Consider keeping a journal to write down your thoughts and feelings, and practice mindfulness meditation to help you stay in the present moment.

By recognizing your stressors and understanding how they affect you, you can learn to better manage them and reduce your stress levels. With practice, you can become your own therapist and take control of your mental health.

# Observe Your Feelings and Thoughts

Being your own therapist can be a daunting task. It requires self-awareness, self-reflection, and a willingness to take responsibility for yourself. It also requires a commitment to learning and practicing techniques that can help you manage your feelings and thoughts.

The first step in being your own therapist is to observe your feelings and thoughts.

This means being mindful of your emotions and how they affect your behavior. Pay attention to when you feel overwhelmed, anxious, angry, or sad. Notice your thoughts, too. What kind of thoughts comes up when you're feeling a certain emotion? Are they helpful? Are they negative?

The next step is to identify any patterns in your feelings and thoughts. Are there any common themes? Are there any unhealthy ways of thinking or behavior that you need to address?

Once you have identified your feelings and thoughts, you can begin to figure out how to manage them. This can involve developing coping strategies, such as deep breathing, journaling, or talking to a friend. Or it could involve exploring new ways of thinking, such as cognitive-behavioral therapy or mindfulness.

Finally, you can use the insights you've gained from your observations to create new habits and behaviors. For example, if you've noticed that you're often anxious in certain situations, you can practice relaxation techniques or take time to reflect on how to approach the situation differently.

Being your own therapist takes time and effort, but it can be a rewarding experience. By observing your feelings and thoughts and identifying patterns, you can create healthier habits and start to take control of your life.

## Develop Self-Compassion

Self-compassion is a powerful tool for personal growth and well-being. It is the ability to recognize and accept our imperfections and weaknesses, while also being kind and understanding toward ourselves. It can help us to be more self-aware and to make better choices that will ultimately lead to greater happiness and fulfillment.

Self-compassion requires us to be both patient and honest with ourselves. We must be willing to forgive ourselves for our mistakes and to recognize and accept our vulnerabilities. We must be able to give ourselves space to make mistakes and to learn from them without judging ourselves.

When we practice self-compassion, we become more resilient in the face of life's challenges. We become more accepting of ourselves and are better equipped to handle difficult situations. We gain self-assurance and comfort in our own skin.

There are numerous methods for learning self-compassion. One way is to practice mindfulness, which is the practice of being present at the moment and observing our thoughts and feelings without judgment. This helps us to become more self-aware and to recognize our needs and limitations. Another way to develop self-compassion is to practice self-care. This means making time for ourselves and engaging in activities that make us feel good, such as getting enough sleep, eating healthy, exercising, and taking breaks from our work. We can also practice self-care by taking time to journal, meditate, or do something creative.

We can also practice self-compassion by learning to be kinder to ourselves. We can practice self-talk and affirmations, which are positive statements that we can say to ourselves to remind us of our strengths and to motivate us to take steps toward our goals.

Developing self-compassion is an important part of becoming our own therapist. It helps us to be more understanding and accepting of ourselves and to make better decisions in our lives.

# Establish Self-Care Practices

Self-care is an important practice for mental health and well-being. It involves taking steps to ensure that your physical and psychological needs are met, while also creating a space where you can be in tune with your emotions and thoughts. Establishing self-care practices can be an effective way to become your own therapist and manage your mental health. The first step in establishing self-care practices is to identify your needs. This can be done by reflecting on what activities make you feel most relaxed, energized, and content. This could be anything from journaling, going for a walk, or listening to music. Once you have identified your needs, you can begin to create a routine for yourself. This routine could include setting aside time each day to engage in activities that meet your needs.

Next, it is important to create an environment that is conducive to self-care. This could involve creating an environment that is free from distractions, such as setting aside time for yourself away from screens or noise. It could also involve creating a comfortable space that is free from clutter and organized in a way that is conducive to mental health and relaxation.

It is important to practice self-compassion and self-awareness. This involves being mindful of your thoughts and feelings and responding to them in a kind and understanding way. It also involves being aware of your limitations and setting realistic goals for yourself.

Overall, establishing self-care practices can be an effective way to become your own therapist and manage your mental health. It involves identifying your needs, creating a routine, and creating an environment that is conducive to self-care. Additionally, it involves practicing self-compassion and self-awareness. With the right approach, you can be your own therapist and take steps to improve your mental health and overall well-being.

# Chapter 4

## Steps to Self-Therapy

1. Acknowledge your feelings: Recognize your emotions and how they are impacting your life. Understand that it's okay to feel whatever you are feeling and that it's a normal part of the human experience.

2. Identify the underlying cause: Search for the root cause of your distress. Take a

step back and ask yourself questions to identify the source.

3. Examine your thoughts: Reflect on the thoughts that are contributing to your distress. Are they based on facts or assumptions? Are they helping or hurting?

4. Create a plan of action: Develop a plan for addressing your feelings and thoughts. Consider methods such as cognitive-behavioral therapy and mindfulness.

5. Take small steps: Break down your plan into manageable tasks. Start with small steps and build upon them until you reach your goals.

6. Monitor your progress: Track your progress and monitor your progress.

Recognize areas where you can tweak things or improve.

 7. Reach out for help: Seek out the support of friends and family or find a therapist who can help you with more challenging issues.

8. Make self-care a priority: Take care of yourself and your physical and mental health. Regular exercise, a balanced diet, and relaxation exercises are all recommended.

 9. Celebrate your successes: Celebrate the successes and acknowledge the progress you have made. This will help to motivate you to continue on your journey.

10. Practice gratitude: Develop an attitude of gratitude and appreciation for the life you have. This will help to create a sense of inner peace and joy.

# Assessing Your Mental Health

Assessing your mental health is an important step in taking care of yourself. It can be helpful to monitor your mental health on a regular basis and implement healthy coping strategies to maintain a positive outlook. There are several ways to assess your mental health and be your own therapist.

First, be aware of your thoughts and feelings. Pay close attention to how your thoughts and feelings affect you. Notice if your thoughts are helping or hindering you. If they are causing you distress or worry, try to develop healthier thoughts that are more positive and supportive. Second, keep track of your moods and behaviors. This can help you identify any patterns that might be affecting your mental health. Consider keeping a journal or diary of your daily activities, including your thoughts and feelings. This can help you recognize any changes in your mental health over time.

Third, make sure you are getting enough sleep and taking care of your physical health. Make sure to get adequate sleep and consume a healthy diet. Exercise can also be beneficial for your mental health, as it can help reduce stress and anxiety.

Fourth, practice relaxation and mindfulness techniques. Look for relaxing activities you can do, like yoga, meditation, or deep breathing. These activities can help you manage stress and anxiety and can help you be more aware of your thoughts and feelings.

Finally, reach out for support when needed. Talk to a friend or family member about your feelings and any struggles you might be experiencing. If you feel like you need professional help, consider talking to a mental health professional.

Assessing your mental health and being your own therapist is an important step in taking care of yourself. Pay attention to your thoughts and feelings, take care of your physical health, and reach out for help when needed. Implementing these strategies can help you stay mentally healthy and maintain a positive outlook.

# Understanding Your Feelings and Thoughts

Understanding your feelings and thoughts is an important part of being your own therapist. Being able to recognize, understand and process your feelings and thoughts is vital for mental health and well-being.

Start by identifying your feelings and thoughts. Be aware of what you are feeling and thinking at any given moment. Consider asking yourself: How am I feeling right now? What am I thinking about? What emotions am I experiencing? This can help you become more aware of your feelings and thoughts.

Once you have identified your feelings and thoughts, it's important to understand why you are feeling and thinking the way you do. Consider asking yourself: What caused this emotion? What thoughts led to this feeling? What could be the source of my current feelings? This can help you gain insight into your emotions and thoughts.

Next, it's important to process your feelings and thoughts. Ask yourself questions such as: What can I do to make this feeling go away? What is a healthy approach for me to deal with this? What can I do to move forward? This will help you find positive ways to manage your emotions and thoughts.

Finally, it's important to learn from your feelings and thoughts. Consider the following: What can I learn from this experience? What can I do differently next time? What can I do to prevent this feeling from returning? This can help you build resilience and become more aware of your emotions and thoughts in the future.

Understanding your feelings and thoughts is an important part of being your own therapist. By recognizing, understanding, and processing your feelings and thoughts, you can gain insight into your mental health and well-being.

# Developing Coping Mechanisms

Coping mechanisms are the strategies and behaviors people use to manage stress and cope with difficult situations. Developing coping mechanisms can help you deal more effectively with life's challenges and become your own therapist.

One way to develop coping mechanisms is to recognize the signs of stress and recognize when you need to take a break. Acknowledge when you are feeling overwhelmed and practice self-care. This may include activities such as deep breathing, yoga, or going for a walk. Taking a break can help you process your thoughts and feelings.

Another approach to developing coping mechanisms is to practice mindfulness. This involves paying attention to your thoughts and feelings in the present moment without judgment. It can help you gain insight into how you think and act and can also help you develop healthier coping skills.

Another way to develop coping mechanisms is to identify your triggers. Understanding what triggers your stress and anxiety can help you find ways to prevent it from happening in the future. This may involve avoiding certain people or situations that may cause you to stress. Finally, it's important to practice self-compassion. Be kind to yourself and recognize that mistakes are part of life. Acknowledge your own strengths and weaknesses and practice positive self-talk. This can help you build resilience and cope more effectively with challenging situations.

Developing coping mechanisms is an important part of self-care. By learning to recognize your own triggers, practice mindfulness, and be kind to yourself, you can become your own therapist and develop the skills to manage stress and difficult situations.

# Creating a Self-Care Plan

Creating a self-care plan is essential for taking care of your mental and physical health. A self-care plan will help you to better manage stress, practice healthier habits, and identify what triggers difficult emotions. By taking the time to create a self-care plan, you can begin to practice self-care in a more mindful and intentional way.

The first step to creating a self-care plan is to identify your needs. Think about the areas of your life that you would like to improve or enhance. Consider areas like physical health, mental health, spiritual health, financial health, social health, and emotional health. Make a list of the things you want to focus on and make sure to include activities that help you to relax, reduce stress, and boost your mood.

The next step is to create actionable goals. Decide on specific goals that you want to focus on, such as exercising for 30 minutes each day or making time for relaxation. Once you have your goals, create a plan for achieving them. Consider what activities and resources you need to make it happen. When creating your plan, be sure to include activities that bring you joy.

Finally, it's important to assess and reassess your self-care plan regularly. Make sure that it's meeting your needs and that it's helping you to achieve your goals. As your life changes, so should your self-care plan. Be sure to adjust it as needed in order to keep it up to date. Creating a self-care plan can help you to practice self-care in a more intentional and mindful way. It can help you to better manage stress and practice healthier habits. Make sure to include activities that bring you joy and assess your plan regularly to ensure that it's meeting your needs.

# Chapter 5

# Ways of Maintaining Self-Therapy

Maintaining self-therapy is a powerful tool for achieving personal growth, as it helps you identify and address difficulties in your thoughts, emotions, and behaviors.

There are various ways to practice self-therapy, and they include being mindful, practicing self-compassion, setting boundaries, and engaging in self-care. Being mindful is a form of self-therapy that involves being aware of your thoughts and feelings in the present moment. This can help you identify and address negative thought patterns or unhealthy behaviors. Practicing self-compassion is another way to maintain self-therapy, as it involves treating yourself with kindness and understanding. It can help you recognize and accept your flaws and vulnerabilities. Setting boundaries is an important part of self-therapy, as it helps you establish healthy relationships with yourself and others. This involves setting limits and expectations for yourself and others and learning to stand up for yourself when necessary.

Engaging in self-care is a great way to practice self-therapy. Self-care involves taking time to do activities that nourish your mind, body, and soul. Examples of self-care activities include exercise, meditating, journaling, spending time in nature, and pursuing hobbies or interests. These are just a few of the ways you can practice self-therapy. By being mindful, practicing self-compassion, setting boundaries, and engaging in self-care, you can create a healthier relationship with yourself and work towards achieving personal growth.

# Journaling

Journaling is a powerful tool for self-exploration and reflection and can be a great way to be your own therapist. It can help you to identify and process your feelings, gain clarity and insight, take steps towards personal growth, and better understand yourself.

When journaling, it's important to make sure you're comfortable and in a relaxed environment. Make sure that you have plenty of time to journal without interruption. It's also important, to be honest with yourself and to write without judgment.

Start by focusing on the present moment and writing down your thoughts and feelings, without overthinking them. Try to be descriptive and explore your feelings more deeply. You may find that it helps to write down questions to explore, such as 'What is making me feel this way?' or 'What is the root cause of this emotion?' Journaling can also be a great way to explore potential solutions or ways of coping with difficult emotions. Writing down different coping strategies and seeing how they work in practice can help you to find the ones that work best for you.

You can also use journaling to set goals and plan out steps to achieve them. Writing down your goals and breaking them down into small, achievable steps can help to keep you motivated and on track.

Journaling can be an incredibly therapeutic and healing activity. Give it a try and see how it can help you to be your own therapist.

# Seeking Professional Guidance

Seeking professional guidance can be a valuable tool in managing your mental health. Being your own therapist can help you gain insight into yourself, recognize patterns in your behavior, and develop new approaches to self-care. It can be a great way to take control of your mental health and create a healthier lifestyle.

The first step in seeking professional guidance on how to be your own therapist is to identify your goals and determine what type of help you need. Do you need help with managing stress, dealing with depression, or coping with difficult emotions? Knowing these types of questions can help you find the best therapist for your needs.

Once you have identified your goals, it's important to find a professional who is experienced in helping people be their own therapists. Many therapists are familiar with self-help techniques, so it's important to ask about their experience and training. It's also a good idea to find out if the therapist offers telehealth services if that's an option for you.

During your sessions, the therapist will help you identify the underlying issues that are causing your mental health struggles. This can be difficult work, and it might be uncomfortable at times, but it's essential for making lasting changes. The therapist will work with you to develop a plan of action that is tailored to your individual needs.

Once you've identified the underlying issues, it's important to work on developing new habits and approaches to self-care. This may include learning relaxation techniques, exploring mindfulness, or journaling. The therapist can help you identify which techniques are best suited to your needs.

By working with a professional, you can learn how to be your own therapist. This can be a powerful tool in managing your mental health and creating a healthier lifestyle.

# Connecting with Others

Connecting with others can be a powerful tool in becoming your own therapist. Having a strong support system of friends and family can provide a sense of comfort and understanding, as well as help to normalize experiences and provide insight into different perspectives. Talking to someone you trust about your thoughts and feelings can help to reduce the intensity of distressing emotions, which can in turn help to create clarity and provide different perspectives.

When it comes to being your own therapist, connecting with others can also be a great way to get more information and expand your own knowledge. For example, talking to a trusted friend or family member who has gone through a similar experience can provide insight into how they were able to cope and can provide you with additional resources. Additionally, talking to a professional therapist can provide guidance and support in navigating difficult emotions, as well as help to gain insight into your own thought processes and behaviors.

Connecting with others can also help to create a sense of safety and acceptance, which can help to reduce the sense of isolation and loneliness. By having meaningful conversations and connecting with others, we can feel less alone in our experiences and gain the courage to take on difficult emotions. Additionally, connecting with others can also be a great way to practice self-care. For example, taking time for yourself to be with friends, or spending time with family can be a great way to take a break from your own thoughts and feelings.

Overall, connecting with others can be a powerful tool in how to be your own therapist. By connecting with those around us, we can gain insight, receive support, and create a sense of safety and acceptance. Additionally, we can gain the courage to face difficult emotions and learn more about ourselves. Ultimately, connecting with others can be a great way to get the help you need and practice self-care.

# Conclusion

Congratulations! You have completed an important step in taking control of your mental health. You now have the necessary tools and knowledge to conduct your own therapy sessions. Your journey doesn't end here, however. With continued effort and dedication, you can continue to build upon the skills and knowledge you have developed in order to maintain a healthy mental state. Remember that self-therapy is a practice that requires regular commitment and effort. You are the only one who can decide to create and sustain a healthy and balanced lifestyle. Take the time to reflect on what you have learned, and be sure to revisit your notes and resources to stay on track. With persistence and resilience, you can achieve a more stable and improved mental state. Good luck in your journey to self-discovery!

www.ingramcontent.com/pod-product-compliance
Lightning Source LLC
Chambersburg PA
CBHW051829250726
48659CB00005B/1751